Starting a Dog Breeding Business

Step by Step How to Get Money, Supplies & Equipment

By Brian Mahoney

DEDICATION

**This book is dedicated to my son's
Christian and Matthew.
A blessing from God and the joy of my life.**

ACKNOWLEDGMENTS

I WOULD LIKE TO ACKNOWLEDGE ALL THE HARD WORK OF THE MEN AND WOMEN OF THE UNITED STATES MILITARY, WHO RISK THEIR LIVES ON A DAILY BASIS, TO MAKE THE WORLD A SAFER PLACE.

Disclaimer

This book was written as a guide to starting a business. As with any other high yielding action, starting a business has a certain degree of risk. This book is not meant to take the place of accounting, legal, financial or other professional advice. If advice is needed in any of these fields, you are advised to seek the services of a professional.

While the author has attempted to make the information in this book as accurate as possible, no guarantee is given as to the accuracy or currency of any individual item. Laws and procedures related to business are constantly changing.

Therefore, in no event shall Brian Mahoney, the author of this book be liable for any special, indirect, or consequential damages or any damages whatsoever in connection with the use of the information herein provided.

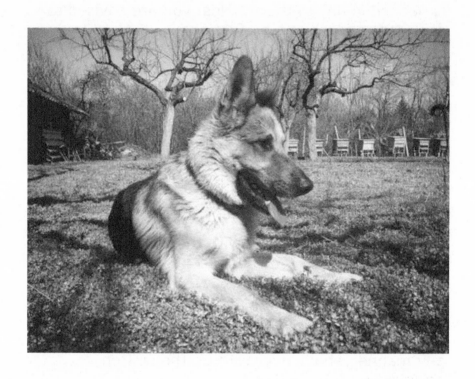

Table of Contents

Chapter 1

Dog Breeding

Overview

DOG BREEDING

American Dog Breeders Association

The American Dog Breeders Association, Inc. was started in September, 1909 as a multiple breed association. The residing president, Mr. Guy McCord, was an avid fancier and breeder of the American Pit Bull Terrier, and was a close friend of Mr. John P. Colby. Mr. Colby was the mainstay of the A.D.B.A. which prompted the boast of being the "home" registration office of the Colby dogs. All members, in good standing, could register their dogs and litters with the registration department upon the yearly payment of $2.50 dues fee. It seems that the exclusive member's idea gradually was replaced into an open registry to all owners and breeders of purebred dogs. Over time the association became focused on the registration of the American Pit Bull Terrier.

Dog Breeding Overview

The A.D.B.A. passed from the hands of Mr. McCord to Mr. Frank Ferris in 1951. He, along with his wife Florence Colby, (the wife of the late John P. Colby) continued to run the A.D.B.A. on a limited scale, but with ever increasing emphasis on the registration of the A.P.B.T. breed exclusively.

In 1973, through the recommendation of Howard Heinzl, Ralph Greenwood and his family purchased the A.D.B.A. from Mr. Ferris, whose advancing age prompted his retirement. (Mr. Heinzl was a personal friend of Frank Ferris and a staunch supporter of the A.D.B.A., as he registered his dogs exclusively with A.D.B.A.) We often wish Frank could have lived to witness the growth of the present association. He would have been pleased.

The association continues to grow in the USA and other countries overseas. The American Dog Breeders Association Inc. is the largest registration office of the American Pit Bull Terrier and now accepting other purebred dogs, usually working breeds.

Beginning 27 October 2006 the registry is opening its stud book to accept other purebred dogs.

Dog Breeding Overview

What is Dog breeding?

Dog breeding is the practice of mating selected dogs with the intent to maintain or produce specific qualities and characteristics. When dogs reproduce without such human intervention, their offsprings' characteristics are determined by natural selection, while "dog breeding" refers specifically to the artificial selection of dogs, in which dogs are intentionally bred by their owners. A person who intentionally mates dogs to produce puppies is referred to as a dog breeder. Breeding relies on the science of genetics, so the breeder with a knowledge of canine genetics, health, and the intended use for the dogs attempts to breed suitable dogs.

Dog Breeding Overview

History

Three generations of "Westies" in a village in Fife, Scotland

Humans have maintained populations of useful animals around their places of habitat since pre-historic times. They have intentionally fed dogs considered useful, while neglecting or killing others, thereby establishing a relationship between humans and certain types of dog over thousands of years. Over these millennia, domesticated dogs have developed into distinct types, or groups, such as livestock guardian dogs, hunting dogs, and sighthounds. Artificial selection in dog breeding has influenced behavior, shape, and size of dogs for the past 14,000 years.

The evolution of dogs from wolves is an example of neoteny or paedomorphism selection, that results in a retention of juvenile physical characteristics. Compared to wolves, many adult dog breeds retain such juvenile characteristics as soft fuzzy fur, round torsos, large heads and eyes, ears that hang down rather than stand erect, etc.; characteristics which are shared by most juvenile mammals, and therefore generally elicit some degree of protective and nurturing behavior cross-species from most adult mammals, including humans, who term such characteristics "cute" or "appealing".

Dog Breeding Overview

It has been seen that these traits can even prompt an adult female wolf to act more defensively of dog puppies than of wolf puppies. The example of canine neoteny goes even further, in that the various dog breeds are differently neotenized according to the type of behavior that was selected.

To maintain these distinctions, humans have intentionally mated dogs with certain characteristics to encourage those characteristics in the offspring. Through this process, hundreds of dog breeds have been developed. Initially, the ownership of working and, later, purebred dogs, was a privilege of the wealthy. Nowadays, many people can afford to buy a dog. Some breeders chose to breed purebred dogs, while some prefer the birth of a litter of puppies to a dog registry, such as kennel club to record it in stud books such as those kept by the AKC (American Kennel Club).

Such registries maintain records of dogs' lineage and are usually affiliated with kennel clubs. Maintaining correct data is important for purebred dog breeding. Access to records allows a breeder to analyze the pedigrees and anticipate traits and behaviors.

Dog Breeding Overview

Requirements for the breeding of registered purebreds vary between breeds, countries, kennel clubs and registries. It has been concluded that "findings imply that when selective breeding was done by humans, it squashed the snouts of certain dog breeds, it also morphed their brains" (Scientific American, 2010). Breeders have to abide by the rules of the specific organization to participate in its breed maintenance and development programs. The rules may apply to the health of the dogs, such as joint x-rays, hip certifications, and eye examinations; to working qualities, such as passing a special test or achieving at a trial; to general conformation, such as evaluation of a dog by a breed expert. However, many registries, particularly those in North America, are not policing agencies that exclude dogs of poor quality or health. Their main function is simply to register puppies born of parents who are themselves registered.

Dog Breeding Overview

Criticism

Some dogs have certain inheritable characteristics that can develop into a disability or disease. Canine hip dysplasia is one such condition. Some eye abnormalities, some heart conditions, and some cases of deafness have been proven to be inherited. There have been extensive studies of these conditions, commonly sponsored by breed clubs and dog registries, while specialised breed clubs provide information of common genetic defects for their breeds. As well, special organizations, such as Orthopedic Foundation for Animals, collect data and provide it to breeders, as well as to the general public. Conditions such as hip dysplasia can impact some breeds more than others.

Some registries, such as American Kennel Club, may include a record of the absence of certain genetic defects, known as a certification, in an individual dog's record. For example, the German Shepherd Dog national breed club in Germany is a registry that recognizes that hip dysplasia is a genetic defect for dogs of this breed.

Dog Breeding Overview

Accordingly, it requires all dogs to pass evaluation for absence of hip dysplasia to register their progeny, and records the results in individual dog's pedigrees.

There are BBC documentaries titled "Pedigree Dogs Exposed" and "Pedigree Dogs Exposed – Three Years On" that claim health problems in dogs from inbreeding. Problems such as breathing in the Pug breed and Pekingese breed, spinal problems in the Dachshund breed, and Syringomyelia in the Cavalier King Charles Spaniel breed.

Some scientific researchers argue that advances in artificial reproduction technology for the purposes of dog breeding can be helpful but also have "detrimental impacts" when overused instead of natural selection principles. These scientists call for a deeper understanding of natural selection, leading to a more naturalistic approach in dog breeding.

Dog Breeding Overview

Purebred dog

A purebred dog typically refers to a dog of a modern dog breed with a documented pedigree in a stud book and may be registered with a breed club that may also be part of a national kennel club.

Purebred dog may also be used in a different manner to refer to dogs of specific dog types and landraces that are not modern breeds. An example is cited by biologist Raymond Coppinger, of an Italian shepherd who keeps only the white puppies from his sheep guardian dog's litters, and culls the rest, because he defines the white ones as purebred. Coppinger says, "The shepherd's definition of pure is not wrong, it is simply different from mine." However, the usual definition is the one that involves modern breeds.

Registration

Purebred dogs are pedigreed members of modern breeds. These dogs may be registered with breed club. The breed clubs may be an open stud book or a closed stud book, the term can be interpreted to either. Usually the breed club is also associated with a kennel club (AKC, UKC, CKC etc.). However dogs who are registered with a breed club are usually referred to as "registered".

Dog Breeding Overview

Some use the term exclusively for a dog that has also been registered with a breed club, but more often it is used simply as a generic term to refer to dogs who have known pedigrees within a standardized breed. A dog that is purebred cannot be interpreted to mean it is high-quality dog. It is no reflection on the quality of the dog's health, temperament or sagacity, but merely a reference that the dog has known parentage according to the breeder. While some breed clubs can now guarantee parentage through DNA testing for the most part all breed clubs must rely exclusively on the breeder's word and choice of parentage. In the early years of the kennel club concept this was not at issue since dog breeding was only done among the extremely wealthy and their reputations were at stake. However in this modern age of breeding one must be aware that even a DNA proven purebred and registered champion who has won national competitions can have serious health issues.

Dog Breeding Overview

The closed stud book requires that all dogs descend from a known and registered set of ancestors; this results in a loss of genetic variation over time, as well as a highly identifiable breed type, which is the basis of the sport of conformation showing. In order to enhance specific characteristics, most modern purebred dogs registered with closed stud books are highly inbred, increasing the possibility of genetic-based disease.

The open stud book, meaning some outcrossing is acceptable, is often used in herding dog, hunting dog, and working dog (working dog meaning police dogs, assistance dogs, and other dogs that work directly with humans, not on game or livestock) registries for dogs not also engaged in the sport of conformation showing. Outcrosses with other breeds and breeding for working characteristics (rather than breeding for appearance) are assumed to result in a healthier dog. Overuse of one particular stud dog due to the desirability of the dog's working style or appearance leads to a narrowing of genetic diversity, whether the breed uses an open stud book or a closed stud book.

Dog Breeding Overview

The Jack Russell Terrier Club of America states, "Inbreeding favors genes of excellence as well as deleterious genes." Some open stud book breeds, such as the Jack Russell Terrier, have strict limitations on inbreeding.

Dog Crossbreeds

Dog crossbreeds (first generation crosses from two purebred dogs, also called dog hybrids) are not breeds and are not considered purebred, although crossbreds from the same two breeds of purebreds can have "identical qualities", similar to what would be expected from breeding two purebreds, but with more genetic variation. However, crossbreds do not breed true (meaning that progeny will show consistent, replicable and predictable characteristics), and can only be reproduced by returning to the original two purebred breeds.

Among breeds of hunting, herding, or working dogs in open stud book registries, a crossbred dog may be registered as a member of the breed it most closely resembles if the dog works in the manner of the breed.

Dog Breeding Overview

Some hunting, herding, or working dog registries will accept mixed breed (meaning of unknown heritage) dogs as members of the breed if they work in the correct manner, called register on merit.

Mixed Breed

For mixed breed (unknown heredity), crossbred (from two different purebred breeds), or otherwise unregistered purebred pet dogs there are available many small for-pay internet registry businesses that will certify any dog as a purebred anything one cares to invent.

However, new breeds of dog are constantly being legitimately created, and there are many websites for new breed associations and breed clubs offering legitimate registrations for new or rare breeds. When dogs of a new breed are "visibly similar in most characteristics" and have reliable documented descent from a "known and designated foundation stock" they can then be considered members of a breed, and, if an individual dog is documented and registered, it can be called purebred. Only documentation of the ancestry from a breed's foundation stock determines whether or not a dog is a purebred member of a breed.

Dog Breeding Overview

Showdog

The term showdog is commonly used in two different ways. For people in the dog fancy, a showdog is an exceptional purebred dog that conforms to breed type, and an outgoing, high energy character. For people who have no interest in dog shows, the term "showdog" is often used facetiously to refer to a dog whose only attributes are in its appearance. Raymond Coppinger says, "This recent breeding fad for the purebred dog is badly out of control.".

Dog shows (and the related sport of Junior Handling for children and young people) continue to be popular activities; a single show, the 2006 Crufts dog show alone had 143,000 spectators, with 24,640 purebred dogs entered, representing 178 different breeds from 35 different countries. The sport of conformation dog showing is only open to registered purebred dogs.

Dog Breeding Overview

Health issues

Genetic conditions are a particular problem for dogs from registries whose stud books are closed. Many national kennel clubs prohibit registering dogs that have or carry certain genetic illnesses. Some of the most common conditions include hip dysplasia, seen in large breed dogs, von Willebrand disease, a disease that affects platelets that is inherited in Doberman Pinschers, entropion, a curling in of the eyelid seen in Shar Peis and many other breeds, progressive retinal atrophy, inherited in many breeds, deafness, and epilepsy, known to be inherited in Belgian Shepherd Dogs, German Shepherd Dogs, Cocker Spaniels, and St. Bernards. In 2008, the BBC ran a documentary on the health problems in pedigree dogs.

Dog Breeding Overview

Future of purebred dogs

Most Kennel Club breeds that exist today were chosen from existing land-race breeds in the late 19th century. How those dogs appear now however have been customized to fit within the breed club's chosen description of them. To do this, required selective breeding and rigorous culling. This created a genetic bottleneck that some people think will render breeding from closed stud books not viable. Suggestions for improvement have included outcrossing (opening studbooks) and measuring and regulating inbreeding. There are some breeders who take care to ensure that the dogs they breed have not been bred to too many other dogs so that the genetic pool does not shrink from everyone breeding to a popular sire. There are a great deal that are merely breeding two "papered" dogs assuming that is all they need to do.

However, science continues to get better and enables breeders to test for genetic diseases. Where breeders were only able to detect afflicted animals in the past, now DNA tests can be run and only animals without affected genes can be bred to produce stronger breeds.

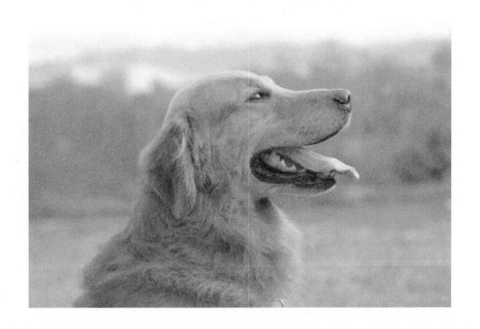

Chapter 2

Dog Breeding

Supplies

& Equipment

Dog Breeding Supplies & Equipment

Pet Edge

PetEdge is a leading supplier of wholesale grooming supplies and discount pet products.

Pet Edge gives you access to over 12,000 national-brand and exclusive PetEdge-brand products through their catalogs and website.

http://goo.gl/R9DDto

ValleyVet

Whether you're looking for prescription medication, vaccines, parasite control, fencing materials, tack, a new pair of boots or anything in between, look no further than ValleyVet who offfer over 23,000 products!

https://urlzs.com/hh2ro

Dog Breeding Supplies & Equipment

Exodus Breeders

Exodus Breeders offer reproductive supplies like

- Insemination kits

- Blood collection supplies

- Canine express semen transport

- Kennel management & supplies

- Ovulation kits and detector

- All plastic steril syringes and needles

- Puppy resuscitator kit

- Semen collection supplies

- Semen freezing management supplies

and much much more!

https://www.exodusbreeders.com/

Dog Breeding Supplies & Equipment

A to Z vet supply

A to Z vet supply has over 50,000 products. Save on everything you need for dog breeding when you buy dog breeding supplies direct from A to Z Vet Supply. They make it affordable and convenient to stock up on quality grooming products, medications, bedding and other kennel supplies.

A to Z Vet Supply is also your one stop resource for whelping supplies, from breeding supplements to pregnancy testing to vaccines for the puppies.

They also offer:

- Flea and Tick control products
- D-Wormers
- Collars and Leases
- Supplements / Nutritional products
- Training aids
- Toys and Treats
- ID systems

https://urlzs.com/kYMf1

Dog Breeding Supplies & Equipment

Complete list of recognized dog breeds

American Kennel Club

The American Kennel Club is dedicated to upholding the integrity of its Registry, promoting the sport of purebred dogs and breeding for type and function. Founded in 1884, the AKC® and its affiliated organizations advocate for the purebred dog as a family companion, advance canine health and well-being, work to protect the rights of all dog owners and promote responsible dog ownership.

Not only can you get a list of all recognized dog breeds but from this web sit you can:

- Get dog training products and services

- Find puppies

- Shop new products

- Get involved in sporting events

- Regisgter your dog

http://www.akc.org/dog-breeds/

Dog Training Supplies

http://www.dog-training.com/

http://www.roverpet.com/

http://www.dogsupplies.com/

http://www.petwholesaler.com/index.php

http://www.happytailsspa.com/

http://www.futurepet.com/

http://www.petmanufacturers.com/

http://www.k9bytesgifts.com/

http://www.kingwholesale.com/

http://www.upco.com/

CERTIFICATION PROGRAMS

Certification Council for

Professional Dog Trainers

The Certification Council for Professional Dog Trainers® (CCPDT®) is the leading independent testing and certification resource for dog training and behavior professionals. They set the global standard for the development of rigorous exams to demonstrate mastery of humane, science-based dog training practices. They are a private, not-for-profit organization.

http://www.ccpdt.org/

The Association of

Professional Dog Trainers

Whether you are just embarking on a dog training career, a seasoned industry veteran, or just trying to decide how best to add a dog to your family, the APDT is where you will find the advice, support, and training you need.

https://apdt.com/join/certification/

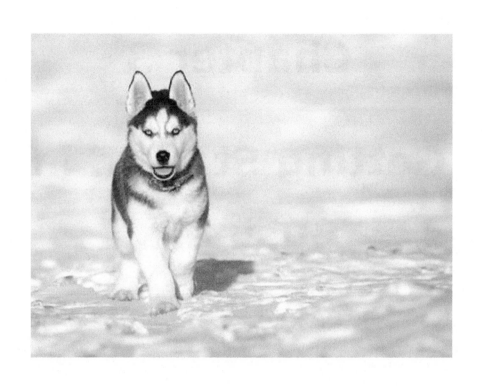

Chapter 3

Getting Started in Business

Step by Step

Getting Started in Business

There are over thirty million home-based businesses in the United States alone.

Many people dream of the independence and financial reward of having a home business. Unfortunately they let analysis paralysis stop them from taking action. This chapter is designed to give you a road map to get started. The most difficult step in any journey is the first step.

Anthony Robbins created a program called Personal Power. I studied the program a long time ago, and today I would summarize it, by saying you must figure out a way to motivate yourself to take massive action without fear of failure.

2 Timothy 1:7 King James Version

"For God hath not given us the spirit of fear; but of power, and of love, and of a sound mind."

Getting Started in Business

STEP #1 MAKE AN OFFICE IN YOUR HOUSE

If you are serious about making money, then redo the man cave or the woman's cave and make a place for you to do business, uninterupted.

STEP #2 BUDGET OUT TIME FOR YOUR BUSINESS

If you already have a job, or if you have children, then they can take up a great deal of your time. Not to mention well meaning friends who use the phone to become time theives. Budget time for your business and stick to it.

STEP #3 DECIDE ON THE TYPE OF BUSINESS

You don't have to be rigid, but begin with the end in mine. You can become more flexible as you gain experience.

STEP #4 LEGAL FORM FOR YOUR BUSINESS

The three basic legal forms are sole proprietorship, partnership, and corporation. Each one has it's advantages. Go to www.Sba.gov and learn about each and make a decision.

STEP #5 PICK A BUSINESS NAME AND REGISTER IT

One of the safest ways to pick a business name is to use your own name. By using your own name you don't have to worry about copy right violations.

However, always check with an Attorney or the proper legal authority when dealing with legal matters.

STEP #6 WRITE A BUSINESS PLAN

This would seem like a no brainer. No matter what you are trying to accomplish you should have a blueprint. You should have a business plan. In the NFL about seven headcoaches get fired every season. So in a very competetive business, a man with no head coaching experience got hired by the NFL's Philadelphia Eagles. His name was Andy Reid. Andy Reid would later become the most successful coach in the team's history. One of the reasons the owner hired him, was because he had a business plan the size of a telephone book. Your business plan does not need to be nearly that big, but if you plan for as much as possible, you are less likely to get rattled when things don't go as planned.

STEP #7 PROPER LICENSES & PERMITS

Go to city hall and find out what you need to do, to start a home business.

STEP #8 PUT UP A WEB SITE, SELECT BUSINESS CARDS, STATIONERY, BROCHURES

This is one of the least expensive ways to not only start your business but to promote and network your business.

STEP #9 OPEN A BUSINESS CHECKING ACCOUNT

Having a separate business account makes it much easier to keep track of profit and expenses. This will come in handy, whether you decide to do your own taxes or hire out an professional.

STEP #10 TAKE SOME SORT OF ACTION TODAY!

This is not meant to be a comprehensive plan to start a business. It is meant to point you in the right direction to get started. You can go to the Small Business Administration for many free resources for starting your business. They even have a program(SCORE) that will give you access to many retired professionals who will advise you for free! Their web site: **www.score.org**

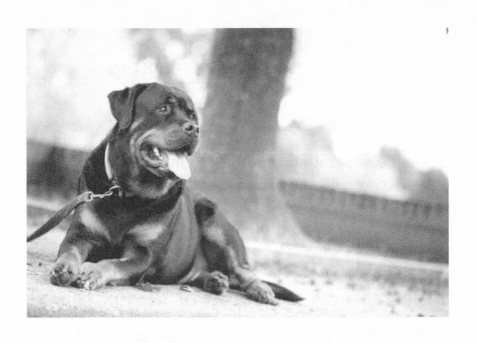

Chapter 4
Best Way
To Write A
Business Plan

How to Write a Business Plan

Millions of people want to know what is the secret to making money. Most have come to the conclusion that it is to start a business. So how do you start a business? The first thing you do to start a business is to create a business plan.

A business plan is a formal statement of a set of business goals, the reasons they are believed attainable, and the plan for reaching those goals. It may also contain background information about the organization or team attempting to reach those goals.

A professional business plan consists of eight parts.

1. Executive Summary

The executive summary is a very important part of your business plan. Many consider it the most important because this part of your plan gives a summary of the current state of your business, where you want to take it and why the business plan you have made will be a success. When requesting funds to start your business, the executive summary is a chance to get the attention of a possible investor.

2. Company Description

The company description part of your business plan gives a high level review of the different aspects of your business. This is like putting your elevator pitch into a brief summary that can help readers and possible investors quickly grasp the goal of your business and what will make it stand out, or what unique need it will fill.

3. Market Analysis

The market analysis part of your business plan should go into detail about your industries market and monetary potential. You should demonstrate detailed research with logical strategies for market penetration. Will you use low prices or high quality to penetrate the market?

4. Organization and Management

The Organization and Management section follows the Market Analysis. This part of the business plan will have your companies organizational structure, the type of business structure of incorporation, the ownership, management team and the qualifications of everyone holding these positions including the board of directors if necessary.

5. Service or Product Line

The Service or Product Line part of your business plan gives you a chance to describe your service or product. Focus on the benefits to the customers more than what the product or service does. For example, a air conditioner makes cold air. The benefit of the product is it cools down and makes customers more comfortable whether they are driving in bumper to bumper traffic or are sick and sitting in a nursing home. Air Conditioners fill a need that could mean the difference between life and death. Use this section to state what are the most important benefits of your product or service and what need it fills.

6. Marketing and Sales

Having a proven marketing plan is a essential element to the success of any business. Today online sales are dominating the marketplace. Present a strong internet marketing plan as well as social media plan. YouTube videos, Facebook Ads and Press Releases all can be part of your internet marketing plan. Passing out flyers and business cards are still an effective way to reach potential customers.

Use this part of your business plan to state your projected sales and how you came to that number. Do your research on similar companies for possible statistics on sales numbers.

7. Funding Request

When you write your Funding Request section of your business plan, be sure to be detailed and have documentation of the cost of supplies, building space, transportation, overhead and promotion of your business.

8. Financial Projections

The following is a list of the important financial statements to include in your business plan packet.

Historical Financial Data

Your historical financial data would be bank statements, balance sheets and possible collateral for your loan.

Prospective Financial Data

The prospective financial data section of your business plan should show your potential growth within your industry, projecting out for at least the next five years.

You can have monthly or quarterly projections for the first year. Then project from year to year.

Include a ratio and trend analysis for all of your financial statements. Use colorful graphs to explain positive trends, as part of the financial projections section of your business plan.

How to Write a Business Plan

Appendix

The appendix should not be part of the main body of your business plan. It should only be provided on a need to know basis. Your business plan may be seen by a lot of people and you don't want certain information available to everybody. Lenders may need such information so you should have an appendix ready just in case.

The appendix would include:

Credit history (personal & business)

Resumes of key managers

Product pictures

Letters of reference

Details of market studies

Relevant magazine articles or book references

Licenses, permits or patents

Legal documents

Copies of leases

Building permits

Contracts

List of business consultants, including attorney and accountant

Keep a record of who you allow to see your business plan.

Include a Private Placement Disclaimer. A Private Placement Disclaimer is a private placement memorandum (PPM) is a document focused mainly on the possible downsides of an investment.

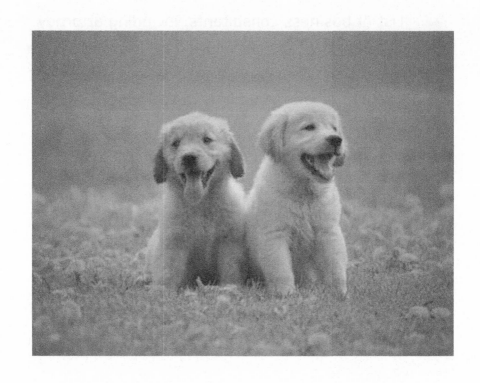

CHAPTER 5
Business
Insurance

BUSINESS INSURANCE

Consult an attorney for any and all of your business matters.

In the early 1990's an elderly woman purchased a hot cup of coffee from a McDonald's drive-thru window in Albuquerque. She spilled the coffee, and suffered 3rd degree burns. She sued Mcdonald's and won. She won 2.7 million dollars in a punitive damages victory. The verdict was appealed and settlement is estimated at somewhere in the neighborhood of $500,000 dollars. All because she spilled the coffee into her lap, while trying to add sugar and cream.

Two men in Ohio, were carpet layers. They were severely burned when a three and a half gallon container of carpet adhesive ignited, when the hot water heater it was sitting next to, was turned on. They felt the warning lable on the back of the can was insufficient. So they filed a lawsuit against the adhesive manufacturers and were awarded nine million dollars.

A woman in Oklahoma, purchased a brand new Winnebago. While driving it home, she set the cruise control to 70 miles per hour. She then left the drivers seat to make some coffee or a sandwich in the back of the motor home.

BUSINESS INSURANCE

The vehicle crashed and the woman sued Winnebago for not advising her, that cruise control does not drive and steer the vehicle. She won 1.7 million dollars and the company had to rewrite their instruction manual.

Unfortunately all three outrageous lawsuits are real. If you are going to run a business, any business, you should consider protecting yourself with Professional Liability Insurance, also known as Errors and Omissions (E & 0) insurance.

This type of insurance can help to protect you from having to pay the full cost of defending yourself against a negligence lawsuit claim.

Error and Omissions can protect you against claims that are not usually covered in regular liability insurance. Those policies usually cover bodily harm, or damage to property. Error and Omissions can protect you agaist negligence, and other mental anguish like inaccurate advice, or misrepresentation. Criminal prosecution is not covered.

Errors and Ommision insurance is recommended for notaries public, real estate brokers or investors and professionals like: software engineers, lawyers, home inspectors web site delvelopers and landscape architects to name a few professions.

BUSINESS INSURANCE

The Most Common Errors and Omission Claims:

%25 Breach of Fiduciary Duty

%15 Breach of Contract

%14 Negligence

%13 Failure to Supervise

%11 Unsuitability

%10 Other

BUSINESS INSURANCE

Things you should know about or require before purchasing a Errors and Omission policy is...

* What is the limit of liability

* What is the Deductible

* Does it include FDD First Dollar Defense - which obligates the insurance company to fight a case without a deductible first.

* Do I have Tail-end coverage or Extended Reporting Coverage (insurance that lasts into retirement)

* Extended coverage for Employees

* Cyber Liability Coverage

* Department of Labor Fiduciary Coverage

* Insolvency Coverage

If you get Errors and Omission insurance, renew it the day it expires. You must be careful to avoid gaps in your coverage, or it could result in not getting your policy renewed.

BUSINESS INSURANCE

A few E & O Insurance Providers:

Insureon

Insureon states that their median Errors and Omissions Insurance policy cost about $750 a year or about $65 a month. The price of course will vary according to your business, the policy you choose and other risk factors.

https://www.insureon.com/home

EOforless

EOforless.com helps insurance, investment, and real estate professionals buy E & O insurance at an affordable cost in five minutes or less.

https://www.eoforless.com/

BUSINESS INSURANCE

CalSurance Associates

As a leading insurance broker, CalSurance Associates, a division of Brown & Brown Program Insurance Services, Inc. has over fifty years of experience delivering comprehensive insurance products, exceptional service, and proven results to over 150,000 insured. They provide professionals nationwide and across multiple industries, including some of the largest financial firms and insurance companies in the United States.

http://www.calsurance.com/csweb/index.aspx

Better Safe Than Sorry

Insurance is one of the hidden costs of doing business. These are just a few companies and a brief overview on the topic of business insurance. Make sure to talk to an attorney or quailified insurance agent before making any decision on insurance. Protect you and your business. Many states do not require E & O insurances. But when you see the cost of some of the settlements, it's better to be safe than sorry.

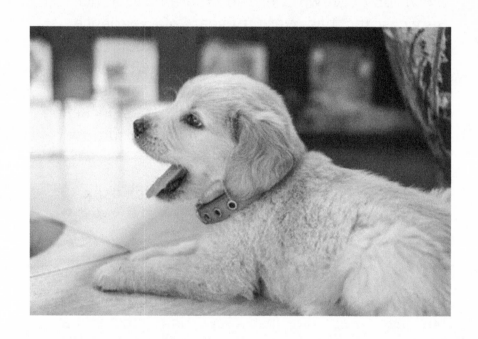

Chapter 6

Goldmine of Government Grants

How to write a Winning Grant Proposal

Goldmine of Government Grants

Government grants. Many people either don't believe government grants exist or they don't think they would ever be able to get government grant money.

First lets make one thing clear. Government grant money is **YOUR MONEY**. Government money comes from taxes paid by residents of this country. Depending on what state you live in, you are paying taxes on almost everything....Property tax for your house. Property tax on your car. Taxes on the things you purchase in the mall, or at the gas station. Taxes on your gasoline, the food you buy etc.

So get yourself in the frame of mind that you are not a charity case or too proud to ask for help, because billionaire companies like GM, Big Banks and most of Corporate America is not hesitating to get their share of **YOUR MONEY**!

There are over two thousand three hundred (2,300) Federal Government Assistance Programs. Some are loans but many are formula grants and project grants. To see all of the programs available go to:

https://beta.sam.gov/help/assistance-listing

WRITING A GRANT PROPOSAL

The Basic Components of a Proposal

There are eight basic components to creating a solid proposal package:

1. The proposal summary;

2. Introduction of organization;

3. The problem statement   (or needs assessment);

4. Project objectives;

5. Project methods or design;

6. Project evaluation;

7. Future funding; and

8. The project budget.

WRITING A GRANT PROPOSAL

The Proposal Summary

The Proposal Summary is an outline of the project goals and objectives. Keep the Proposal Summary short and to the point. No more that 2 or 3 paragraphs. Put it at the beginning of the proposal.

Introduction

The Introduction portion of your grant proposal presents you and your business as a credible applicant and organization.

Highlight the accomplishments of your organization from all sources: newspaper or online articles etc. Include a biography of key members and leaders. State the goals and philosophy of the company.

The Problem Statement

The problem statement makes clear the problem you are going to solve(maybe reduce homelessness). Make sure to use facts. State who and how those affected will benefit from solving the problem. State the exact manner in how you will solve the problem.

WRITING A GRANT PROPOSAL

Project Objectives

The Project Objectives section of your grant proposal focuses on the Goals and Desired outcome.

Make sure to indentify all objectives and how you are going to reach these objectives. The more statistics you can find to support your objectives the better. Make sure to put in realistic objectives. You may be judged on how well you accomplish what you said you intended to do.

Program Methods and Design

The program methods and design section of your grant proposal is a detailed plan of action.

What resources are going to be used.

What staff is going to be needed.

System development.

Create a Flow Chart of project features.

Explain what will be achieved.

Try to produce evidence of what will be achieved.

Make a diagram of program design.

WRITING A GRANT PROPOSAL

Evaluation

There is product evaluation and process evaluation. The product evaluation deals with the result that relate to the project and how well the project has met it's objectives.

The process evaluation deals with how the project was conducted, how did it line up with the original stated plan and the overall effectiveness of the different aspects of the plan.

Evaluations can start at anytime during the project or at the project's conclusion. It is advised to submit a evaluation design at the start of a project.

It looks better if you have collected convincing data before and during the program.

If evaluation design is not presented at the beginning that might encourage a critical review of the program design.

Future Funding

The Future Funding part of the grant proposal should have long term project planning past the grant period.

WRITING A GRANT PROPOSAL

Budget

Utilities, rental equipment, staffing, salary, food, transportation, phone bills and insurance are just some of the things to include in the budget.

A well constructed budget accounts for every penny.

For a complete guide for government grants google

catalog of federal domestic assistance. You can download a complete PDF version of the catalog.

Other sources of Government Funding

You can get General Small Business loans from the government. Go to the Small Business Administration for more information.

SBA Microloan Program

The Microloan program provides loans of up to $50,000 with the average loan being $13,000.

https://www.sba.gov/

WRITING A GRANT PROPOSAL

Recently billionaire Elon Musk was awarded 4.9 billion dollars in government subsidies. If you are hesitant to pursue government assistance, let that sink in. A billionaire who pays little in taxes was given billions of your tax dollars.

Government grants are real. Like anything else worthwhile, there is effort and qualifications that must be met to obtain them.

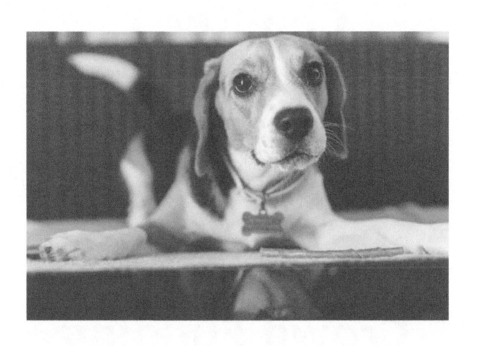

Chapter 7

Colossal Cash

from

Crowd Funding

Crowd Funding Crowd Sourcing

In 2015 over $34 billion dollars was raised by crowdfunding. Crowdfunding and Crowdsourcing roots began in 2005 and they help to finance or fund projects by raising money from a large number of people, usually by using the internet.

This type of fundraising or venture capital usually has 3 components. The individual or organization with a project that needs funding, groups of people who donate to the project, and a organization sets up a structure or rules to put the two together.

These websites do charge fees. The standard fee for success is about %5. If your goal is not met there is also a fee.

Below is a list of the top Crowdfunding websites according to myself and Entrepreneur Magazine Contributor Sally Outlaw.

Crowd Funding Crowd Sourcing

https://www.indiegogo.com/

Started as a platform for getting movies made, now helps to raise funds for any cause.

http://rockethub.com/

Started as a platform for the arts, now it helps to raise funds for business, science, social projects and education.

http://peerbackers.com/

Peerbackers focuses on raising funds for business, entrepreneurs and innovators.

https://www.kickstarter.com/

The most popular and well know n of all the crowdfunding websites. Kickstarter focuses on film, music, technology, gaming, design and the creative arts. Kickstarter only accepts projects from the United States, Canada and the United Kingdom.

Crowd Funding Crowd Sourcing

Group Growvc

http://group.growvc.com/

This website is for business and technology innovation.

https://microventures.com/

Get access to angel investors. This website is for business startups.

https://angel.co/

Another website for business startups.

https://circleup.com/

Circle up is for innovative consumer companies.

https://www.patreon.com/

If you start a YouTube Channel (highly recommended) you will hear about this website frequently. This website is for creative content people.

Crowd Funding Crowd Sourcing

https://www.crowdrise.com/

"Raise money for any cause that inspires you."
The Landing page slogan speaks for itself. #1
fundraising website for personal causes.

https://www.gofundme.com/

This fundraising website allows for business, charity,
education, emergencies, sports, medical, memorials,
animals, faith, family, newlyweds etc...

https://www.youcaring.com/

The leader in free fundraising. Over $400 million
raised.

https://fundrazr.com/

FundRazr is an award-winning online fundraising
platform that has helped thousands of people and
organizations raise money
for causes they care about.

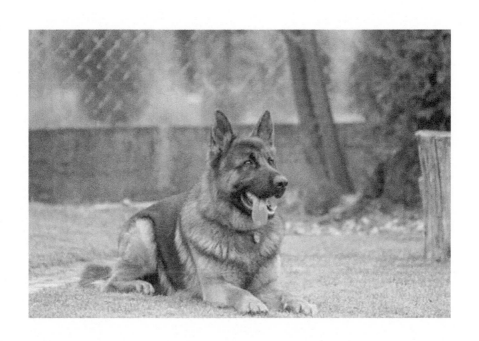

Chapter 8

Marketing How To Reach a Billion People for Free!

How to Reach a Billion People for Free!

Marketing your coffee shop business is essential to it's success. In today's business environment marketing does not have to be expensive. With social media and big search engines like Google and YouTube you can get your business in front of millions of people with out it costing a fortune.

ZERO COST MARKETING

While there are many ways to market we are only going focuse on ZERO COST MARKETING. You are starting up. You can always go for the more expensive ways of marketing after your business is producing income.

FREE WEB HOSTING

Get a free web site. You can get a free web site at weebly.com or wix.com. Or just type "free web hosting" in a google, bing or yahoo search engine.

Free web hosting is something you can use for a varitey or reasons. However many free web hosting sites add an extention to the name of you web address that lets everyone know you are using their services. For this reason you eventually want to scale up once you start making income.

How to Reach a Billion People for Free!

LOW COST PAID WEB HOSTING

Free is nice, but you when you need to expand your business it is best to go with a paid web hosting service. There are several that give you good value for under $10.00 a month.

1. Yahoo small business

2. Intuit.com

3. ipage.com

4. Hostgator.com

5. Godaddy.com

Yahoo small business allows for unlimited web pages and is probably the best overall value, but they require a years payment up front. Intuit allows for monthly payments.

For free ecommerce on your web site, open up a Paypal account and get the HTML code for payment buttons for free. Then put those buttons on your web site.

How to Reach a Billion People for Free!

Step 1 zero cost internet marketing

Now that your web site is up and running you should register it with at least the top 3 search engines. 1. Google 2. Bing 3. Yahoo.

Step 2 zero cost internet marketing

Write and submit a **press release**. Google "free press release sites" for press release sites that will allow you to summit press releases for free. I you do not know how to write a press release go to www.fiverr.com and sub-contract the work out for only $5.00 !!!

Step 3 zero cost internet marketing

Write and submit articles to article marketing web sites like **ezinearticles.com.**

Step 4 zero cost internet marketing

Create and submit videos to video sharing sites like dailymotion.com or **youtube.com.** Make sure to include a hyperlink to your website in the description of your videos.

Step 5 zero cost internet marketing

Submit your web site to **dmoz.org**. This is a huge open directory that many smaller search engines go to get web sites for their database.

How to Reach a Billion People for Free!

YouTube has over a billion users. You may already have a YouTube channel and be good at making videos. However if you are not familiar with getting videos made and uploaded to YouTube you can go to a website called....

fiverr

https://www.fiverr.com/

https://goo.gl/R9x7NU

https://goo.gl/B7uF4L

https://goo.gl/YZ6VdS

https://goo.gl/RoPurV

At fiverr you can get a YouTube video created quickly and easily for only $5.00.
        (currently there is also a $1 service fee)

So for less than a movie ticket you can have a commercial for your real estate or business running 24 hours a day 7 days a week.

Once the video is uploaded you need to know how to get people to view your video. That's where SEO search engine optimization comes in.

How to Reach a Billion People for Free!

Getting Your Video Seen

YouTube reads any interaction that the viewer takes with your video as a sign that your video is interesting. So a Thumbs up or like will boost the ranking of your video.

Viewer comments can boost a video in the search rankings. So one tip for getting a viewer to leave a comment is to say "I'm curious what do you think about (insert topic). Another way to get viewer comments is to create a video about gun control laws, race relations, abortion rights or any other controversial topic.

YouTube can send a notice to all of your Subscribers every time you upload a video. So the more subscribers you have, the better chance that your video will get views, and views help the rank the video higher in the YouTube search results.

Getting your viewer to share a link to their social media pages is what makes our video go viral. Great or entertaining content is the key. It also does not hurt to simply ask the viewer to do it.

Rather than say the same thing every video, you can create a "close" video and upload it to YouTube. Then you can use the YouTube editor to add it to any video you upload.

How to Reach a Billion People for Free!

Search Engine Optimization (SEO) is the term used for the techniques used to drive traffic to your video. Many people use tactics that are against YouTube rules to drive traffic to their videos. These are call "Black Hat". There are plenty of web sites where you can purchase views to your videos. I would advise that you stay away from any possible unethical tactics. Get your views organically.

You can start your video off with good traffic, by sending it in a link to all the people you email to on a regular basis.

Google Keyword Tool

You begin your SEO by using the Google Keyword Tool. Go to

https://adwords.google.com/KeywordPlanner

Once there you type in your root keyword or keyword phrase. Google will then give you about 700-1200 results that it thinks is relevant to your original keyword or phrase. Selecting the right keywords for your video is the key to being able to rank your videos.

How to Reach a Billion People for Free!

How to Select Your Keywords

Once you have your 700 results you can sort the results by relevance. This will give you a high chance for ranking for the original keyword or phrase that you entered.

You can sort your results by competition. You can chose low competition keywords or phrase to increase your chances of getting ranked. The low competition usually have less "per month" searches, but a combination of a few rankings can sometimes be better that just getting one keyword to rank.

Article Marketing

Ezine Articles is one of the top Article Marketing sites on the internet. You can join for free at http://ezinearticles.com/. Once you join the site you can upload articles to this web site that are relevant to your YouTube video. Ezine allows for you to place a link in your article. The link can go back to your YouTube traffic and dramatically increase the views.

When you write your article you should try to match as much as you can to your YouTube video. Use the same headlines, titles and description, as much as possible. YouTube and Google love relevance.

How to Reach a Billion People for Free!

Your article should be between 700 and 800 words. This is about the size that many blogs prefer. Once your article is uploaded onto Ezine articles, it can be picked up by any web site in the world. I once had an article about marketing photography get picked up by almost 800 blogs around the world. Many of them left the link placed in the article, and that allowed for tons of traffic to be drawn to my videos or web site. Not all blogs are ethical and many will remove your link, to keep traffic on their web site. Many will also replace you link with theirs. You won't know until you try.

Press Releases

One of the most powerful ways to increase traffic to your videos is to write and submit a press release. If you have never written a press release don't be intimidated. Your can go to a website www.fiverr.com and get a press release written for only $5.00!

If you want to write the press release yourself here are some tips.

The basic format is 3 paragraphs on one page, for immediate release. Unless it involves a date like a holiday in which you might want to have the editor delay the release.

How to Reach a Billion People for Free!

The headline should be attention getting. If you don't get the attention of the editor, the rest of the press release will not get read. Go to press release websites and look at press releases that have been published and study the headlines and the proper format.

After you have crafted your headline you write 3 paragraphs. The first paragraph is a short summary of what your story is all about. "But I have so much to tell I can't summarize it in a short paragraph." The revolutionary war has a ton of tremendous stories. Entire 2 hour movies have been made about it. Here is a two sentence description of those events. The future United States colonies fought the British. The colonies won!

Paragraph two is descriptions your story. Keep it in the form of a news story. Do not try to sell in your press release. Entertainment show are good at bringing on a celebrity, making small take, then ending the interview with a pitch or plug for their product or cause...

Paragraph three is your call to action. "For more information about how to help the victims of dipsy-doodle-itis call 555-1212 or hit this link."

Most press release website will allow you to place at least one link in your press release.

How to Reach a Billion People for Free!

Here is a list of the top five free press release websites:

Top Free Press Release Websites

https://www.prlog.org

https://www.pr.com

https://www.pr-inside.com

https://www.newswire.com

https://www.OnlinePRNews.com

How to Reach a Billion People for Free!

Social Media Websites

When you upload your videos to YouTube you should comment and like your own video. Once you like your own video, YouTube will give you the option to link the video to powerful social media websites. So you need to join these websites before you upload your videos. Below is a list of some of the social media websites you should join. When you link your videos to these websites, it creates a backlink to a highly rated website, which in turn factors into YouTube and Google's algorithm of what video is considered relevant and most popular.

Social Media Websites

https://www.facebook.com

https://www.tumbler.com

https://www.pinterest.com

https://www.reddit.com

https://www.linkedin.com/

http://digg.com/

https://twitter.com

https://plus.google.com/

How to Reach a Billion People for Free!

Finally, one of the most successful marketing methods being used today is "Permission Marketing". That is where you get a potential customer to give you their email address, and thus permission to market them.

You need a marketing automation platform and an email marketing service. These companies store and send out your emails.

Getresponse, MailChimp and Aweber are some of the more popular email storage autoresponder companies.

To build up and email list you usually have to offer a free product, report or book in exchange for the email address. Then you send them to a web page that captures and stores the email address. An example of my own email capture page is at the end of this book.

For detailed training videos on this and other marketing training hit the link below.

https://goo.gl/3bsRwg

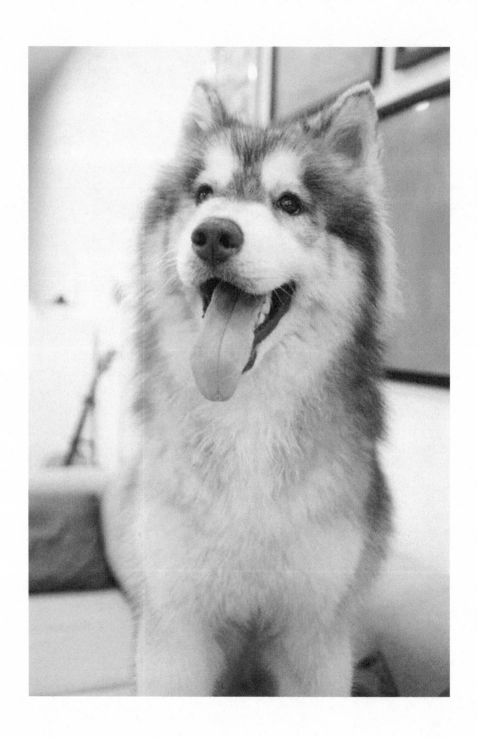

Chapter 9

DOG BREEDING WEB RESOURCE GUIDE

Web Wholesale Resource Rolodex

As of the writting of this book all, of the companies below, website is up and have an active business. From time to time companies go out of business or change their web address. So, instead of just giving you just 1 source I give you plenty to choose from.

Dog Breeding Supplies

http://goo.gl/R9DDto

http://www.valleyvet.com/c/pet-supplies/dog-breeding-supplies.html

http://www.breederssupply.com/

http://www.atozvetsupply.com/Breeder-supplies-s/20.htm

https://www.exodusbreeders.com/

Organizations

http://www.adbadogs.com/p_home.asp

http://www.arba.org/

http://www.iwdba.org/

Complete list of recognized dog breeds

http://www.akc.org/dog-breeds/

Dog Training Supplies

http://www.dog-training.com/

http://www.roverpet.com/

http://www.dogsupplies.com/

http://www.petwholesaler.com/index.php

http://www.happytailsspa.com/

http://www.futurepet.com/

http://www.petmanufacturers.com/

http://www.k9bytesgifts.com/

http://www.kingwholesale.com/

http://www.upco.com/

CERTIFICATION PROGRAMS

http://www.ccpdt.org/

https://apdt.com/join/certification/

Dog Information
www.rainbowridgekennels.com

TRANSPORTATION
Used Trucks/CARS Online

http://gsaauctions.gov/gsaauctions/gsaauctions/

http://www.ebay.com/motors

http://www.uhaul.com/TruckSales/

http://www.usedtrucks.ryder.com/vehicle/VehicleSearch.aspx?
VehicleTypeId=1&VehicleGroupId=3

http://www.penskeusedtrucks.com/truck-types/light-
and-medium-duty/

Parts

http://www.truckchamp.com/

http://www.autopartswarehouse.com/

Bikes & Motorcycles

http://gsaauctions.gov/gsaauctions/aucindx/

http://www.bikesdirect.com/products/used-bikes/?
gclid=CLCF0vaDm7kCFYtDMgodzW0AXQ

http://www.overstock.com/Sports-
Toys/Cycling/450/cat.html

http://www.nashbar.com/bikes/TopCategories_10053_
10052_-1

http://www.bti-usa.com/

http://evosales.com/

COMPUTERS/Office Equipment

http://www.wtsmedia.com/

http://www.laptopplaza.com/

http://www.outletpc.com/

Computer Tool Kits

http://www.dhgate.com/wholesale/computer+repair+t
ools.html

http://www.aliexpress.com/wholesale/wholesale-
repair-computer-tool.html

http://wholesalecomputercables.com/Computer-Repair-Tool-
Kit/M/B00006OXGZ.htm

http://www.amazon.com/Wholesale-Computer-Repair-
Screwdriver-Insert/dp/B009KV1MM0

http://www.tigerdirect.com/applications/category/cate
gory_tlc.asp?CatId=47&name=Computer%20Tools

Computer Parts

http://www.laptopuniverse.com/

http://www.sabcal.com/

other

http://www.nearbyexpress.com/

http://www.commercialbargains.co

http://www.getpaid2workfromhome.com

http://www.boyerblog.com/success-tools

american merchandise liquidators

http://www.amlinc.com/

the closeout club

http://www.thecloseoutclub.com/

RJ discount sales

http://www.rjsks.com/

St louis wholesale

http://www.stlouiswholesale.com/

Wholesale Electronics

http://www.weisd.com/

ana wholesale

http://www.anawholesale.com/

office wholesale

http://www.1-computerdesks.com/

1aaa wholesale merchandise

http://www.1aaawholesalemerchandise.com/

big lots wholesale

http://www.biglotswholesale.com/

More Business Resources

1. http://www.sba.gov/content/starting-green-business

home based businesses

2. http://www.sba.gov/content/home-based-business

3. online businesses

http://www.sba.gov/content/setting-online-business

4. self employed and independent contractors

http://www.sba.gov/content/self-employed-independent-contractors

5. minority owned businesses

http://www.sba.gov/content/minority-owned-businesses

6. veteran owned businesses

http://www.sba.gov/content/veteran-service-disabled-veteran-owned

7.   woman owned businesses

http://www.sba.gov/content/women-owned-businesses

8.   people with disabilities

http://www.sba.gov/content/people-with-disabilities

9.   young entrepreneurs

http://www.sba.gov/content/young-entrepreneurs

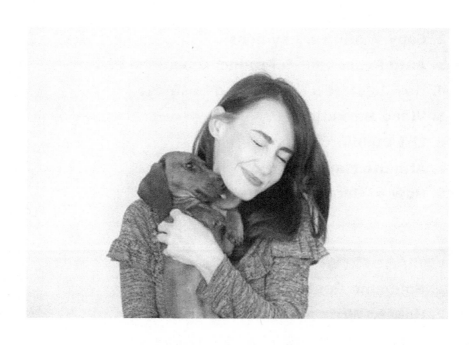

$10,000 MegaSized Internet Marketing &

Copy Writing & SEO Course &

$1,000 Value Bonus

LIBRARY I (Video Training Programs)

1. Product Creation

2. Copy Writing & Payment

3. Auto Responder & Product Download Page

4. How to start a Freelancing business

5. Video Marketing

6. List Building

7. Affiliate Marketing

8. How to Get Massive Web Site Traffic

LIBRARY II (Video Training Programs)

1. Goldmine Government Grants

2. How to Write a Business Plan

3. Secrets to making money on eBay

4. Credit Repair

5. Goal Setting

6. Asset Protection How to Incorporate

$10,000 MegaSized Internet Marketing &

Copy Writing & SEO Course &

$1,000 Value Bonus

Library III

1. SEO SIMPLIFIED PART 1
2. SEO SIMPLIFIED PART 2
3. SEO Private Network Blogs
4. SEO Social Signals
5. SEO Profits

Bonus 1000 Package!

1. Insider Secrets to Government Contracts (PDF)
2. 1000 Books/Guides (text files)
3. Vacation Discounts (text file w/links to discounts)
4. Media Players (3 Software Programs)
100% MONEY BACK GUARANTEE!!!
ALL ON A 8 GIGABYTE FLASH DRIVE

This Massive Library with a $10,000 value all for only a
1 time payment of $67!!!
Get Instant Access by Using the Link Below:

https://urlzs.com/p7v3T

Leave a review and join Our VIP Mailing List Then Get All our Audio Books Free! We will be releasing over 100 money making audio books within the next 12 months! Just leave a review and join our mailing list and get them all for free!

Just Hit/Type in the Link Below

https://urlzs.com/HfbGF

Made in the USA
Las Vegas, NV
06 June 2021